Menopause Explained

Menopause Stages, Perimenopause, Early Menopause, Causes, Symptoms, Treatments, Diet, Health Tips and More!

By Frederick Earlstein

Foreword

The body, in and of itself is a fascinating subject of precision work which has been and is continued to be studied. The reproductive system of a woman is as equally intriguing with all the seeming changes the body of a woman goes through as she matures. There always seem to be something happening that signals one change or another. Here we shall delve into the subject of menopause and discover what every woman needs to know about herself.

Menopause has been a topic that elicits a variety of reactions from many, whether they are men or women. There are many misconceptions that are associated to menopause which we intend to debunk and clarify. We have essentially come up with a handful of important information about what to look out for and expect when dealing with the changes that come with menopause.

This period of change has brought about some of the most fantastic myths and tall stories about what women go through on their way to and upon the onset of menopause. We aim to debunk the misconceptions of this period in a woman's life, as we aim to enlighten the many women who have to go through this period in their lives. As women, we are silently called to be resilient and flexible to changes throughout our lives; you owe it to yourself to do the needful for yourself.

Whatever your conceptions and feelings about menopause, part of your responsibility as a woman, of any age, to take it upon yourself to know what is happening in your body and what to expect as well. The general consensus about menopause can be quite grim - a topic that needs to be talked about in low hushed tones. Although it can be quite daunting to think that your body will actually be going through this process that sounds absolutely horrific, it is not as grim.

As a woman, you want to become proactive when it comes to knowing what you need to learn about your body and the many transitional stages our bodies go through. Your best weapon against the possible health implications brought about by menopause, is to know what your body is going through. Menopause, to a woman unaware of the process can be a crippling blow from a mental perspective.

This stage of a woman's life has enough challenges to one who knows what to expect, it would be mind - blowing to any woman who chooses to keep themselves away from any talk about menopause. The advantages of knowing what to expect, as your body goes through changes, empowers you to take charge of your health and wellbeing. Knowing gives you the chance to find remedies and treatments that are available to you.

Take charge of your life and gain some control over what you can. Find out more about menopause and what you can do to live a better quality of life. Learn about the symptoms, treatments, remedies and ways you can help yourself go and get through what could otherwise be a difficult and lengthy transition.

Table of Contents

Chapter One: Stages of Menopause

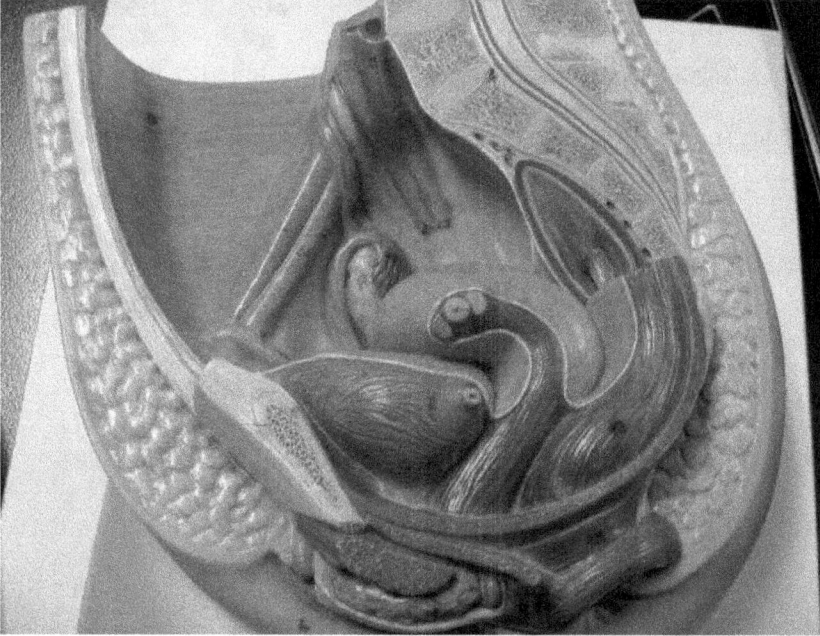

Women go through some of the most amazing body changes as they mature. From the time they are born, their bodies are at work in constant minute and slow transition as it goes through different stages of life. Menopause is another stage of a woman's existence. This is when she ceases to be fertile and monthly menstrual periods have stopped. This is when estrogen levels decrease and ovulation ceases. It can be accompanied by some physical indications in some women and very little symptoms in others. Some women go through night sweat and hot flashes.

Menopause is diagnosed when a woman has not had her period for a span of 12 months. This is not a disease but rather a period in a woman's life when she is no longer fertile, meaning she no longer produces fertile eggs. She no longer ovulates. The time leading up to menopause is called perimenopause. This is a transition period in a fertile woman's life when her body goes through slight and sometimes unnoticeable changes. The symptoms of perimenopause can from two up to ten years to complete and the symptoms for each woman is different. Menopause should be regarded as a positive new stage in a woman's life when she can take the opportunity to take preventative health steps to deter major health risks.

Causes of Menopause

The one major factor that influences menopause is the onset of age. The maturing body of a woman causes the ovaries to slowly lose the ability to manufacture the needed hormones to ovulate. Apart from the natural aging process of a female, there are other factors that can bring about menopause, like medical treatments and surgeries which can bring about early menopause. Some of these situations would include the removal of the ovaries, radiation therapy directed at the pelvis of the female as well as cancer chemotherapy.

A premenopausal woman whose uterus has been removed, or one who undergoes a hysterectomy, appears to have the same symptoms of menopause but the hormonal changes vary slightly. When a woman's uterus is removed through a hysterectomy, without removing her ovaries, her body is no longer able to menstruate, which would cease monthly periods, however, the hormonal changes that comes along with menopause does not occur.

The average age of the onset of menopause is 51. However, menopause can occur in a woman's life later or earlier in their life. There are some women who experience menopause as early as 40 years old. There are also individuals who reach the age of menopause later at the age of 60 years. There seems to be a higher likelihood of women who smoke who experience the onset of menopause earlier than non-smoking women.

Many women wonder when menopause actually begins. There is no surefire way of telling in advance when a woman will reach the age of menopause. This is determined when a woman has noticed that she has not menstruated for 12 consecutive months; the onset of perimenopause to the actual occurrence of menopause usually last anywhere from two to eight years. There are some women who transition quicker than others. The experience is quite different from one woman to the next.

One way of being able to tell, or at least estimate, when you might come into menopause is by finding out when your mother started feeling the symptoms, or perimenopause, to the time she actually experienced her last menstrual period. When your mother started having perimenopause symptoms and when she started menopause can be a good indication of when you will go through menopause.

What is Perimenopause?

The period of transition to menopause up to the period of actual menopause is called perimenopause. This is a period when the estrogen levels in a woman would rise and fall. Perimenopause is when the time nearing menopause commences and the woman may, or may not notice, changes, or "anomalies" in their cycle. During this period, the woman's ovaries are still functioning, but this has notably decreased. It may still be possible for a woman to get pregnant, even with the onset of perimenopausal symptoms. This is because she may still able to ovulate.

Indications of perimenopause vary from woman to woman. It is identified through the noticeable irregularity of the menstrual cycle. Some of the symptoms of perimenopause are the occurrence of hot flashes and tenderness of the breasts. A woman may also notice the worsening symptoms of PMS. She may notice a lower sex drive and feel fatigued. Other indications of perimenopause are vaginal dryness and irregular menstrual periods. She may also notice urine leakage when she coughs or sneezes. A woman may also experience the urgency of urinating.

Women who are going through perimenopause changes would experience mood swings. Some may have trouble sleeping or suffer from interrupted sleep because of other symptoms that may bother their night rests. If a woman is experiencing any of these symptoms, she will want to see her doctor at the soonest possible time because you want to rule out any other conditions, apart from perimenopause, which may be causing these symptoms. You will want to rule out any other conditions that may be causing some, any or all of these indications since it may not be perimenopause which causes these.

Other indications of the possible onset of perimenopause would be heavy periods or periods with blood clots. Periods lasting longer than usual may also be one other indication of the onset of perimenopause as well as spotting instances between periods. In addition, spotting after sex is also another indication of the onset of perimenopause. When periods seem to occur closer to each other, this may also be another indication of the onset of perimenopause.

Indications of Menopause: Period Changes

A woman's menstrual period changes with the approach of menopause. Each woman reports varying degrees of changes. Some woman may experience shorter or longer periods, whilst others notice the changes with lighter or heavier periods. The space between periods may also change noticeably. You may notice an increase or decrease of period frequency. When a woman's body undergoes the initial process of perimenopause, women would notice getting their period after an extended span of no menstrual occurrence.

It is not uncommon for a perimenopausal woman, who has not had her period for a long span, to get her period after several months.

Perimenopausal symptoms can last for years before a woman is actually menopausal. Until a woman has reached a full year of menstrual absence, she may still become pregnant. A woman who notices changes in her menstrual cycle, especially the scarcity of frequency, volume or absence of, should consult with their physician at the soonest possible time because there are other medical conditions which bring about changes in the woman's menstrual cycle.

Around the time of menopause, a woman may begin to notice symptoms of hot flashes. These episodes could be noticed way before menstrual irregularities begin. Hot flashes are manifested with a feeling of warmth which has a tendency to be focused in the neck and face area. Some indications of hot flashes include the reddening of the skin around the face and neck area as well as the back, chest and/or arms. When this happens, hot flashes differ in intensity. Sweating or chills precede hot flashes immediately after the sensation. Waking up at night, drenched in sweat is not unusual and may happen during a hot flush.

Hot flashes are episodes can last for as short as 30 seconds or may last up to 10 minutes. In some women, hot flash episodes may last up to 10 years, however most women (about 80%) will cease to have hot flash episodes after five years of the onset. Why hot flashes happen is an unknown mystery. It is supposed that these episodes are associated to the biochemical and hormonal changes a woman experiences. These could be brought about by lowering estrogen levels.

Hot flashes are thought to occur as a result of the biochemical changes and decreasing estrogen levels of a woman as she matures. It is likely linked to these occurring developments in the changes of the physiology of a woman's body. Women can do a few things to lower the symptoms of hot flashes like exercising regularly; wearing fewer layers of clothes as well as choosing to wear loose-fitting ones could help alleviate the symptoms and severity of hot flashes. Aside from these measures, women can also avoid spicy foods. Eating spicy foods on its own can cause individuals to break out in sweat. Avoiding spicy foods will help lessen the symptoms of hot flash episodes. Managing stress levels is also highly advised to a woman who is undergoing menopausal transition.

Menopause is not a process but a stage in a woman's life when a number of changes occur in her body. It is the period of a woman's life when her ovaries reproductive capacity ends. Menopause is characterized by the woman's absence of menstrual periods in a span of 12 consecutive months. Not every woman will experience all the symptoms of menopause and these signs of menopause may vary from woman to woman. Symptoms of menopause begin to manifest when estrogen levels in the body of a woman decreases.

It is also possible for symptoms of lowered estrogen to manifest years before the actual onset of menopause. The most commonly reported symptoms of menopause include hot flashes and night sweats.

Other symptoms that are associated to the decrease of estrogen levels include vaginal dryness, painful sexual intercourse (dyspareunia). These along with vaginal irritation or itching are reported by and observed in women who are undergoing transitional menopause. An alteration in the urinary system could cause leakage of urine or the need to urinate frequently. Women may experience and notice a bit of urine leakage when they sneeze or cough. Other women report of changes in their skin texture. Some would notice a worsening of acne, or a noticeable weight gain.

Aside from these physical symptoms that manifest the onset of menopause, cognitive and mood shifts can also accompany the onset of menopause in some women. These symptoms vary amongst women. Other symptoms that are associated to menopause are tiredness, fatigue, mood changes, irritability and challenges in memory. Contributing to these cognitive and mental symptoms could be the accompaniment of hot flashes and night sweats which can disrupt sleep patterns and sleep wellness.

Chapter Two: What Women Need to Know

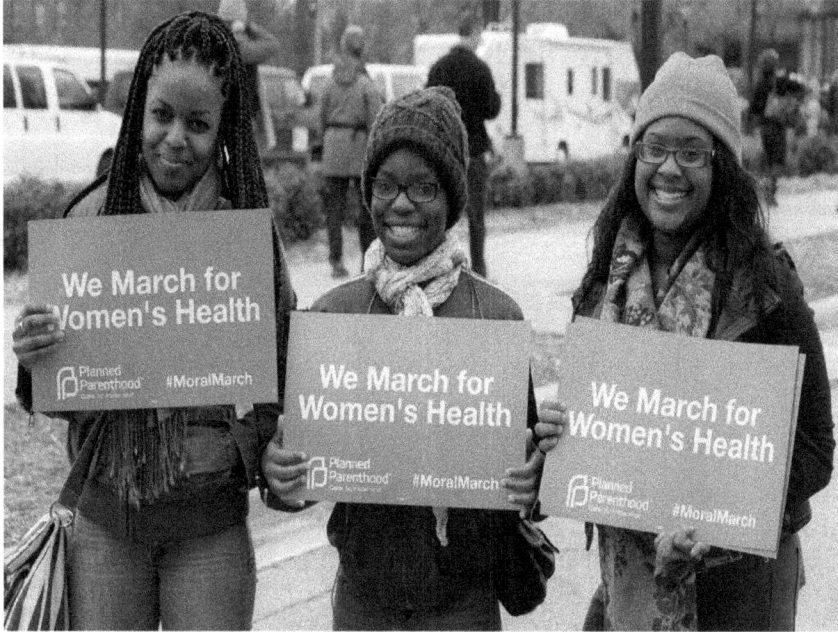

For many women, menopause is a dirty word. It is a topic that most would rather not talk about and something sweeps under the rug, to be dealt with later on. Menopause has been a source of many legendary myths that has given scare to women. Most women would avoid any talk, or give thought, about menopause, pretty much leaving them in the dark as to what to expect and more importantly what she can do. In this chapter, we'll delve deeper regarding what menopause is all about and the things you need to know when it comes to gracefully handling this inevitable phenomenon in every woman's life.

What is Menopause?

Menopause basically is the time when the woman's body ceases to ovulate. It is the stage in her life when she is no longer plagued by the monthly business of having a menstrual period. Like any other milestone in a woman's life, women have to take the proactive approach to menopause to find out what it is about. Menopause is not a process but the time when a woman's period signs off for good. On the other hand, symptoms of menopause actually begin much earlier than most women would care to know. This period of transition is called the perimenopause. This is not an actual medical term, but it is being used more and more to explain the symptoms of menopause and the changes that happen to a woman's body. This is the longer stage of a woman's life when hormonal changes take place.

Perimenopause symptoms vary in intensity and degree in women. Changes in the chemical makeup of the woman take place gradually giving way to symptoms like hot flashes, night sweats, fractured sleep and erratic sleep patterns, a widening of the waistline and a host of other symptoms. Hormonal changes contribute to the bone health of the woman and influence the health of the woman's heart. These can be quite alarming to a woman who has no idea of what to expect as she matures.

Medical experts and practitioners strongly suggest that a woman who is undergoing the transitional changes of perimenopause create healthier habits to help themselves along. There has been strong evidence which reflects that a healthy exercise habit would not only improve a woman's sleep and mood - regular exercise also leads to better blood glucose control, a healthier blood pressure and healthier blood fats.

Exercising does wonders for the immune system which in turn is followed by better health. Where a woman stores her weight in her body can change drastically once she reaches midlife. During her reproductive years, women tend to store surplus fat around their thighs and hips. When menopause comes, a woman would notice that any extra fat she accumulates is stored around her waist area.

This is more than a cosmetic issue since the retention of fat in the abdominal area increases the likelihood of heart disease and type 2 diabetes. This is where, and why, exercise needs to be routine part of a woman's life during this period. All women in their early 30's should get into the habit of exercising before they reach 40, if they can. Women should ideally include strength training to promote stronger bones and to build muscles.

The more muscles a woman develops the less fat she will store. Since muscles burn up more kilojoules than fat does when we are at rest, the more muscles a woman has, the easier it will be for her to keep the extra fat she accumulates in check. As to whether exercise controls or limits the episodes of hot flashes is still a contended debate that needs further studies and research. And this is what was carried out in 2008 by Professor Wendy Brown, from the University of Queensland.

Results of the professor's research had linked weight loss to fewer episodes of hot flashes. Although, exercise does not eliminate the symptoms of menopause, it does greatly help in reducing the discomfort many women who are in the perimenopausal transition, to those in the menopausal stage. Not only has weight loss been linked to a reduction in hot flashes episodes, the study also reflected that weight gain leads to more instances of hot flushes.

Prepare Like a Soldier

The message to women is loud and clear - physical activity and maintaining a healthy weight, sets up women for a leaner and healthier menopause. Menopause should not be something women sweep under the rug only to deal with it later when it is apparent. Like everything else in a woman's life, menopause is something all women, especially those of childbearing age should know about and get ready for.

Maintaining an exercise routine and living a healthy lifestyle early on primes a woman for when she reaches the age of menopause. Having an exercise plan to keep surplus fats at bay and turning them to muscle allows for a mature woman to fare better than one who has not had any preparation for the gradual, sometimes unnoticeable changes menopause brings about in a woman's body.

If you have reached perimenopause and have not had an exercise regimen, now is the time to start. Create some discipline and structure in your life in order to take control of your body and the natural forces of nature. As a woman, you will need to take charge and influence health in your life. There are exercise programs created specifically to target the aim of women in preparation for the onset of menopause.

We all age, however, as individuals, we all have a choice over aging with or without health issues that are preventable. Women, much like soldiers, will have to train to rally on and reap benefits instead of the health challenges that can be brought about by menopause. A combination of cardio and strength training will do wonders for a woman as she goes through the lengthier period of perimenopause as well as lead a healthier lifestyle at the onset of menopause.

Taking action at the earliest possible time in your life can result to a healthier you at sixty than you ever were when you were 30. With many middle-aged women leading more active and productive lifestyles, like working, raising teenagers whilst others are helping out with grandbabies and caring for elderly parents, women are encouraged to take on a bigger role in maintaining better health for a healthier life later.

Chapter Three: What is Early Menopause?

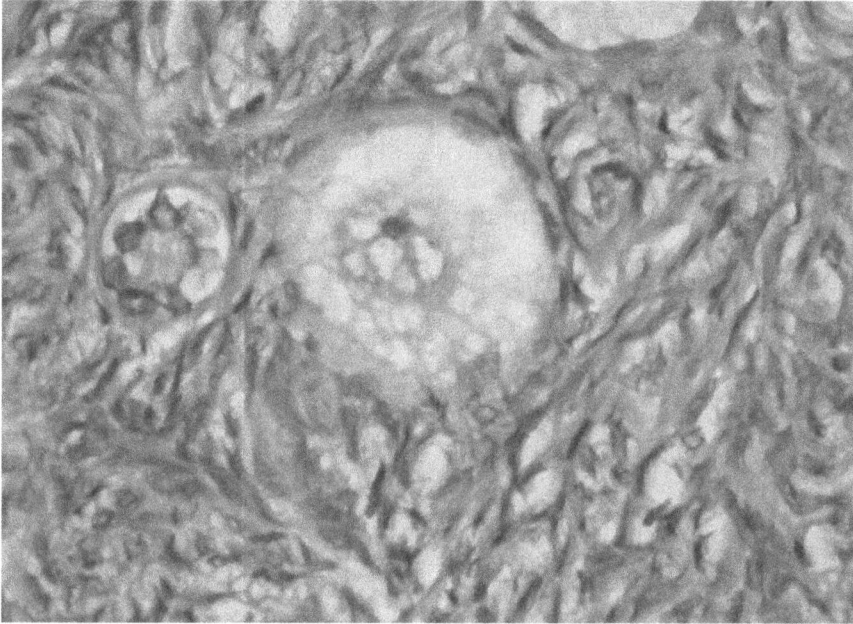

There has been an alarming rise of women going through early menopause, causing great concern with many. With this seeming rise in the number of relatively younger women diagnosed to have reached menopause, further research is needed to come to a reason as to why this is happening. In most cases of premature ovarian failure, there have been no identifiable or concrete causes as of now. However, a small percentage of premature menopauses are due to autoimmune problems and genetic issues.

Early Menopause vs. Premature Menopause

The early occurrence of menopause in younger woman can be due to a number of reasons such as the surgical removal of the ovaries, chemotherapy or radiation treatments that the woman is undergoing as well as the unexplained, premature ovarian failure. Whatever the reason may be, it is important that a woman find out the cause of the early onset of menopause to rule out any underlying, undiscovered condition which may be causing it. This will help moving forward in terms of being given the proper advice by an expert.

Early menopause can come as a shock to a younger woman in her 40's. We typically think, and this is one layman's concept that is supported by medical science, that women reach menopause around 50 to 51 years old. However, there are some women who experience this event earlier in their life. This can be alarming to a woman, who in her 40's would normally be at the prime to give birth.

Early menopause can have a major impact on a woman's well-being, and it may present the woman with a sense of loss or even grief having to experience it younger than expected. It can affect relationships, too because of the decreased sex drive that comes along with it. It has been reported that around 8% of women go through early menopause, and are in the dark about the fact.

The onset of early menopause is defined as the occurrence of the last menstrual period before the woman reaches 45 years old. In some cases of early menopause, there is a likely culprit to blame. It can be brought about by medical treatments like chemotherapy, or by a surgical procedure. However, there are some cases that cannot be explained away by what was mentioned.

Not only is the loss of fertility one consequence of early menopause, the symptoms of menopause can be quite alarming and severe in some cases because of the psychological impacts that come along with the sudden and "unscheduled" changes. This can be quite distressing for a woman, most especially if she is unaware of what is happening to her body. Not only does it affect her ability to bear children, it also opens her up to a host of diseases and conditions which can greatly play on the quality of life she leads.

The sudden change in hormone levels of a woman who has undergone menopause induced by surgery is real as they are sometimes severe and unpredictable. These women tend to have a higher likelihood of developing depression and anxiety. Despite these, early menopause need not be bad news. There are times when the symptoms of menopause outweigh the challenges of having to bear through medical issues that could otherwise be corrected through surgery.

The role of a woman going through the stages of perimenopause and menopause should be one of wanting to be in the know rather than leaving things to chance and, essentially, you in the dark. Be proactive in taking charge of your body and make it your business to know what to expect as you mature. Take the reins and take control of your body, mind and life because menopause is an eventual stage in all women's lives that will happen.

Hormone Replacement Therapy

Hormone replacement therapy, to treat menopause related symptoms like, night sweats, vaginal dryness and hot flashes, continues to be a controversial topic. What was thought to be a drug sent from heaven to relieve women of the bothersome symptoms of menopause, became associated with the increase of breast cancer patients, thereby making use of it take a decline in 2002. However a revisit of the study 10 years after the cessation of research concluded that younger women who used HRT close to the time of menopause resulted in greater benefits when outweighed against the risks.

The commonality of findings resulted in the discovery that HRT and its relation to breast cancer only slightly increased the risk in younger women as opposed to a rise in the oldest candidates included in the decade long research. In conclusion the study that was revisited reflected that women who are found to be at low risk in acquiring breast cancer and who suffer from many of menopausal symptoms may benefit from HRT.

It also appears that a 40% reduction of colorectal cancer in women who used hormone replacement therapy. Aside from this the therapy seems to offer substantial health benefits on the bones which includes a decrease in the risk of fractures. On the other hand, although unfounded and the association not clear yet, the therapy seems to increase the risk of dementia. It is not clear how the risk increase of dementia is related to the age of the woman who is on HRT therapy. In addition, it has been noted that a small increase in the risk of stroke associated with hormone replacement therapy. An increase in the risk of blood clots in the vein or what is medically termed venous thromboembolism.

Chapter Four: Signs and Causes of Early Menopause

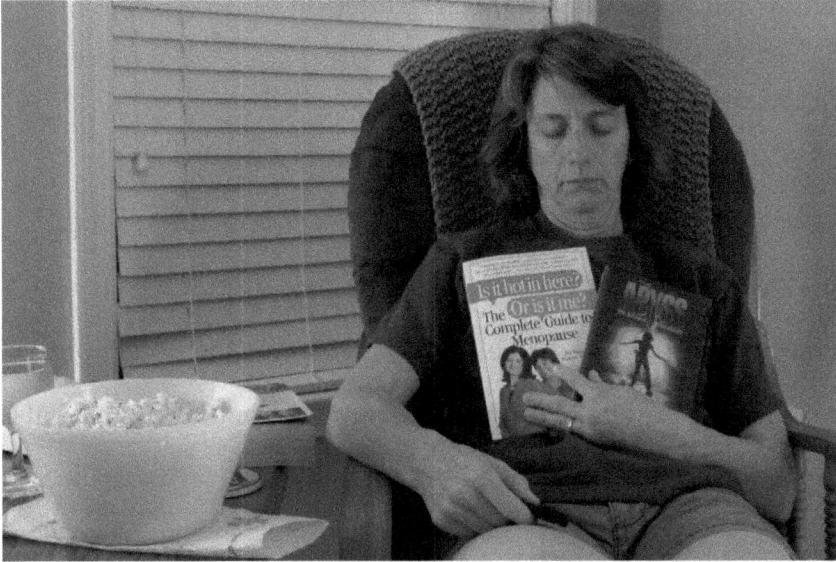

Symptoms of early menopause is not unlike that of regular menopause and some of the symptoms are irregular menstruation cycles, hot flashes accompanied by night sweats, moodiness, mental fogginess, vaginal dryness and a decreased appetite for sex. A woman who has missed having a menstrual period over a period of a few months should consult with her gynecologist immediately as there could be other reasons for the absence of your period such as pregnancy, stress, a change in diet or exercise patterns or an illness. When periods are missed, there is a low level of estrogen and this can lead to bone damage and bone loss. The sooner you know, the sooner you can take action against any bone deterioration and degradation.

Early menopause happens because of follicle dysfunction or follicle depletion. This is a disorder that affects the ability of the ovaries to function as they should and affects about 1% of the female population. This is characterized by low levels of estrogen and the non-occurrence of what should be a woman's regular menstrual cycle.

What is Premature Ovarian Failure?

Premature ovarian failure is defined as the onset of menopause, or one year without menses, before a woman turns the age of 40. This condition is seen in about 1% of all women. To this day, the cause of premature ovarian failure has been a head-scratcher for medical experts and it is still not fully understood. However, there are suspicions that this may be associated with autoimmune diseases or caused by genetic factors.

Premature ovarian failure and premature menopause are not to be confused with each. If the ovaries of a woman cease to function normally before she reaches the age of 40, this is characteristic of premature menopause. Women who have premature ovarian failure may occasionally still experience menstrual periods; however they also usually experience infertility. Premature ovarian failure is usually coupled by primary ovarian insufficiency and has similar symptoms to early menopause. Perhaps due to the age factor, many younger women, with an average age of 40 years old, are experiencing premature menopause and are going undiagnosed. Women who experience premature menopause are at a risk of a number of concerning medical conditions such as dementia, osteoporosis, increased risk of cardiovascular diseases and even premature death.

What makes premature menopause even more alarming is the decrease of the quality of life these women lead because of the early onset of menopause. Conditions ranging from diabetes to rheumatoid arthritis are some of the medical concerns that younger women experience that contribute to a compromised way of living. These conditions make it difficult for women to stay active. Aside from these women who experience the early onset of menopause would also experience hot flashes, night sweats along with mood changes. These are alarming conditions to think about so make it a point to make adjustments.

One out of every 1000 women from ages 15 to 29 are affected with premature ovarian failure and it affects about 1 out of every 100 women who are aged between 30 and 39. Premature ovarian failure can be due to genetic factors that are inherited and passed down, to medical conditions such as eating disorders, thyroid disease, hormonal disorders, autoimmune diseases, and viral infection. The possibilities of having premature ovarian failure increases when a woman is related to people who have gone through the same symptoms; there are also other conditions which may call for the surgical removal the females reproductive parts. Treatment-induced menopause occurs in women who undergo cancer treatments.

How is It Diagnosed?

Your gynaecologist will ask about symptoms you have been experiencing and will inquire about the schedule or cycle of your menstrual period, the occurrence of being around toxins, or if the patient has had to undergo any treatments for cancer. Your OB-GYN may carry out a body examination and may order to have necessary tests done to rule out any other factors.

Your doctor may request to get your blood tested for certain hormones, which would include: follicle-stimulating hormone (FSH), estradiol, and prolactin. On some occasions, your physician may test your DNA for the genetic causes of early or premature menopause.

What Are the Complications?

The chances of a woman developing other conditions such as infertility increases at the onset of early menopause; this can bring about stress and mental anguish as a result from being infertile along with other health issues associated with early menopause. Another complication of early or premature menopause is bone loss (osteoporosis) and this is brought about by low estrogen levels, leaving women more prone to bone degeneration.

Premature Ovarian Failure and You

A disorder which compromises and affects the ovaries to work and do its job as it should is called Premature Ovarian Failure. A small minority of women is affected with premature ovarian failure. POF is also called primary ovarian insufficiency. It is defined by low estrogen levels and missed periods. It could also be symptomatic of autoimmune diseases in women below 40.

On the bright side, POF can be a temporary setback and can be reversed. Those diagnosed with Premature Ovarian Failure may still be able to conceive without fertility intervention. This condition is called ovarian insufficiency, removing the stigma of infertility. The shift in the name of the condition was coined to remove stigma from the younger set of women who undergo early menopause.

It is important to keep in mind that POF and infertility go hand in hand. Women experiencing the absence of their monthly period and who manifest characteristics of infertility could be erroneously diagnosed. When a misdiagnosis is given, the women mistakenly diagnosed would be given recommendation to see a specialist on fertility in order to get prescribed drugs for ovulation. This would not only be an exercise in futility as these drugs don't work on POF. It would only be a waste of time and money and could get the woman's hopes up for an effective treatment to her condition

POF VS Premature Menopause

Menopause is the end of her menstrual life of a woman, is characterized by the absence of menses and normally and naturally happens around the time when a woman reaches 50 years old.

A woman whose final menstrual period occurs before she reaches the age of 40 is called premature menopause. This may happen for two reasons; because of primary ovarian insufficiency or it is brought on as a result of oophorectomy (surgical removal of ovary or ovaries) or cancer treatments such as chemo or radiation therapy.

Premature ovarian failure is not to be mistaken for premature menopause. It is estimated that half the population of women experience this erratic activity and function of the ovary or ovaries for many years. This is why some women get pregnant; it is thought that this is chalked up to misdiagnosis. During treatment of premature ovarian failure replacement of the hormones the body would have normally made on its own is induced through therapy. On the other hand, in the treatment of the symptoms of menopause, focus is trained on extending the hormones and not replacement.

A woman who ceases to menstruate before the age of 40 is defined to be in premature menopause. The causes of premature menopause, when there is no detected cause, are still a mystery but it can stem from a number of reasons as well, like surgery, chemo or radiation treatments. Early menopause is characterized when a woman experiences the last menses before she is 45. Up to 8% of the population of women may experience early menopause and could be induced by surgery, chemo or radiotherapy.

When a woman experiences early menopause, this would mean that she is probably in her mid - 40's and has ceased to menstruate. It is important therefore that a woman who notices irregularities in her menstruation, to discuss this with their health practitioner, namely their gynecologist. There are however, some procedures that a woman may have to go through and treatments she may have to undergo that would bring about premature menopause.

One of these reasons to early menopause is when she has to undergo an oophorectomy. When an ovulating woman has to have her ovaries removed, this will result in an immediate menopause. An oophorectomy, also termed as surgical or induced menopause, will cause the immediate onset of premature menopause. When this is the case, there is no perimenopause stage. The woman who undergoes this sort of induced menopause due to the removal of the ovaries will immediately go through the symptoms of menopause. Most women, however, not all, would frequently say that the sudden onset of the symptoms of menopause can be particularly severe.

During this procedure the ovaries are often removed along with the extraction of the uterus. This is medically called a hysterectomy. When a hysterectomy is done without the extraction of both the ovaries in a woman who has not yet reached menopause, the intact ovary and ovaries will still be capable of the normal hormone production.

While a woman who has undergone a hysterectomy cannot menstruate after the uterus is removed, the ovaries, on their own, manage to continue to manufacture hormones up until the appropriate and normal time when menopause would naturally occur for the woman. During this time, the woman may experience other symptoms of menopause like hot flashes and mood swings. These symptoms would not be related to the cessation of the woman's menstruation and could actually be perimenopause.

Another possibility of premature ovarian failure that takes place earlier than the usual and expected time of menopause (as early as 1 to 2 years) is followed by a hysterectomy. If this were the case, a woman may or may not experience symptoms of menopause. Therefore it is important to communicate your concerns and ask as many questions as you can to your gynecologist.

Cancer Chemotherapy and Radiation Therapy

The type of chemo or radiation therapy and the location treatment is administered can result in the early onset of menopause for an ovulating woman. Depending on the type of cancer and the treatment given, chemotherapy and radiation therapy can bring about almost immediate menopausal symptoms to the woman. When this is the case, the symptoms of menopause could be experienced by the patient during the cancer treatment. On the other hand, symptoms of menopause may also develop in the months following the treatment.

Chapter Five: Causes and Symptoms of Menopause

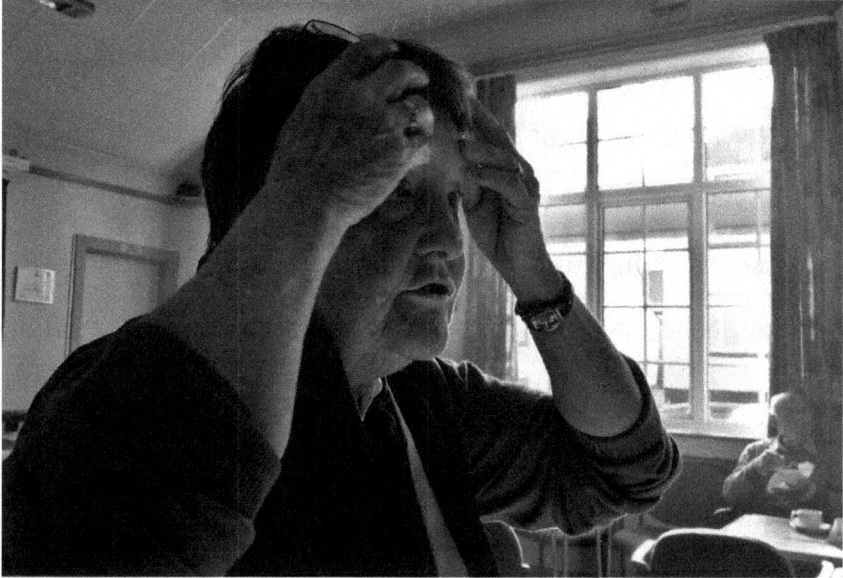

The purpose of finding out symptomatic indications of menopause allows a woman to proactively take charge of her body - and with menopause also having some effect on the moods of a woman, knowing more about the symptoms of menopause allows her to arrest her thoughts before going off the deep end. Empowering yourself should be the first order of business when it comes to things that affect our wellness. A woman, given all the constant and gradual changes her body goes through, should make it her priority to find out about all the possible symptoms she may experience at any given point of transition in her life.

Insomnia is a frequent complaint of women who are undergoing the transitional shifts of menopause. Sleepless nights can be brought about by hot flashes that result in night sweats. These bouts of hot flashes can prevent the woman from having a restful night's sleep. The combination of hot flashes along with uncomfortable sweating can make it very challenging to sleep. The shift's in the levels of a woman's progesterone and estrogen is also another reason for the changes in a woman's sleep quality. To find relief from night sweats, you will want to use light beddings. Use loose fitting clothing to sleep in if you absolutely need to have clothes. Choose materials that are made of cotton and which are lightweight. Make use of a fan in your bedroom (as well as any other room of the house you frequent). You may also want to keep a damp washcloth near your bed. Wiping yourself down will allow your skin to cool down.

Menopause Symptoms

The symptoms of menopause are very different from one woman to the next. Although all women will experience menopause, each woman will go through a personal and unique experience. Each would also have different and varying degrees of the intensity of symptoms. Some women may experience some of the symptoms of menopause that another woman will not, then there are others who will experience a plethora of the symptoms affecting them both in psychological as well as physical levels.

The symptoms of menopause may come and go as they may wane and fade in some women. These symptoms may be noticed for a few months after the last menstruation or it may go on for a few years after the onset.

Irregular Bleeding

Irregular vaginal bleeding is a possibility when a woman reaches menopause. This means that a woman who has ceased to menstruate for a year can experience vaginal bleeding. Some women have very little issues with abnormal bleeding before the prior time to menopause whilst other women experience unpredictable and excessive bleeding during menstrual periods. Menstrual periods, or menses, may happen more frequently; this means that the span of time of the menses is shorter or the menses occur at longer intervals, essentially lengthening the menstrual cycle.

Important Things to Remember

- During perimenopause, there is no way of telling what is typical since menstrual patterns differ with each individual.

- It is not unusual for women who are in perimenopause to experience a period after not having one for several months.

- No one can predict how long the transition to menopause will take.

- A woman can experience irregular periods years prior to her reaching menopause.

- It is important to keep in mind that all women who have irregular menses have to be seen and evaluated by their doctor to determine that the irregular menses are due to perimenopause. The physician will have to rule out other medical conditions.

The abnormalities of a menstrual cycle that starts during the perimenopause stage can be reason for infertility or difficulty in getting pregnant the woman is not able to ovulate properly. On the other hand, perimenopausal women may get pregnant until actual menopause is reached. This can be defined by the absence of menstrual periods for a period of one year. *This can be* defined by the absence of menstrual periods for a period of one year. Therefore, women in the perimenopausal stage should still use contraception if they do not intend to become pregnant.

Night Sweats

Night sweats are defined by episodes of drenching sweats during the nighttime and these are usually accompanied by hot flashes or the feeling of warmth spreading out from your chest, neck and facial regions. This may lead to the abrupt awakening of the individual and the difficulty of falling asleep again. Night sweats can result in a not so refreshing sleep and daytime tiredness.

Hot flashes

Hot flashes are typical complaints and symptoms of menopause. These are bouts of sudden warmth felt throughout, or parts of, the body. It is sometimes related with flushing (redness of skin) and is often times accompanied by sweating. A hot flash episode usually lasts anywhere from 30 seconds up to several minutes. Although the specific reason for hot flashes isn't fully known, they are thought to be caused by the erratic behavior of the hormones.

There is presently no method to foretell when hot flashes will become apparent nor can it be said for sure how long hot flashes will be experienced. These bouts of discomfort are reported by up to 40% of regularly menstruating women in their forties (the perimenopausal period before menopause onset), so they may begin before the menstrual irregularities. An average of about 80% of women will stop experiencing this a few years after the onset.

Occasionally, some women, about 10% of the population, may experience hot flashes longer than others. Some have even reported to experience hot flashes for a decade. In other words, one cannot say for sure when hot flashes will stop, though these episodes have a tendency to lessen in frequency as time passes. They may also wax and wane in their severity. The average woman who has hot flashes will have them for about five years.

Hot flashes are usually accompanied by night sweats; this is when a woman gets drenched in perspiration. Night sweats have been blamed for sudden awakenings in the middle of the night which is accompanied by perspiration. This is why many women who are in the perimenopause, and menopause stages often report poor sleep quality.

Urinary Symptoms

The transport tube beginning at the bladder leading up to discharge urine outside the body, or the lining of the urethra, also experiences the same transformations as the vagina. The urethra becomes drier and less pliable because of the lowering of estrogen levels. This can result bouts of infections in the urinary tract. It may also give the sensation of needing to visit the toilet more. This may also be the reason for leakage of urine, or incontinence. Incontinence is characteristic of a strong, sudden urgency to urinate. Incontinence may also happen when coughing, laughing, or lifting heavy objects.

Vaginal Symptoms

Vaginal symptoms take place because the tissues that line the vagina becomes thinner, drier, and less elastic. The reason for these is due to the estrogen levels that drop. Effects of the symptoms include vaginal dryness, vaginal itching, irritation and/or pain during sexual intercourse, known as dyspareunia. These vaginal changes can also lead to an increased risk of vaginal infections.

Emotional and Cognitive Symptoms

Women who are in the perimenopause transition stage often report of cognitive as well as emotional symptoms which include challenges in recollection or memory problems, fatigue, irritability and sudden shifts in their moods. There is no way of determining and exacting if changes in behavior are related to the erratic changes that accompanies menopause because of many factors that are at play.

Emotional and cognitive symptoms are common that often times it is challenging to determine if the transition to menopause is to blame. Accompanying night sweats that may happen can be contributory to the person being spent. These can greatly factor in in terms of the persons mood and clarity. To top it off, many women may be going through other life shifts during the period of transitional perimenopause or after the onset of menopause; stressful life events are also possible causes of changes and shift in the person's emotions.

Other Physical Changes

Lots of women would notice and often notice an increase in weight during the onset of menopause. The allocation of body fat may change becoming more noticeable in the stomach area and the waist line rather than in the lower extremities and limbs as before the onset of perimenopause or menopause.

The woman would see changes in skin texture. These could include wrinkles, or the worsening of adult acne.

Because the woman is able to manufacture small levels of the male hormone, she could experience minute spurts of hair growing in places she wouldn't normally grow hair, like her upper lip and chin. Some even notice hair growing on their chest and stomach.

Sex Problems

Women in menopause usually have low levels of estrogen hormone; one of the major effects of low estrogen hormones is a decrease of blood supply to the vagina. This causes vaginal dryness, resulting in painful and often times, uncomfortable intercourse. You can solve this problem by using water-soluble lubricants. Should you find that the lubricants you use are not that effective, make an appointment with your doctor and talk about alternative methods they can recommend. Vaginal creams and suppositories may also be prescribed by your doctor to ease the dryness of vagina.

As a woman's body reaches menopausal stage, her body goes through a number of changes. In addition to this, another effect of change in hormones is a shift in sex drive. A woman's libido may either improve or it may worsen. Keep in mind that there are other factors apart from menopause which can affect the woman's libido.

Other factors that can affect the sex drive of a woman are sleeping disturbances, stress, anxiety and medications she may take. Consult with your doctor so that he/she can suggest effective ways of managing the changes in your sex drive, should this happen. Keep in mind that even though menstruation stops already, no matter what age they are, are still susceptible to sexually transmitted diseases; therefore remember to continue practicing safe sex.

Managing Hot Flashes

One requisite of being a woman is finding out about the many changes her body goes through at specific, given times of her life. From the time a girl is born, her body goes through some pretty amazing transitions that she will need to be aware of to get the best out of living. Knowing what to expect long before changes take place allows the more seasoned lady to empower herself into finding out what there is to do for her to be able to make smart decisions about her health and its balance.

One of the more commonly known symptoms of menopause is the occurrence of hot flashes. Hot flashes are described to be incidences when a woman would feel a sudden warmth spread throughout her body, mainly and usually concentrated on the chest, arms, and face regions. Most, but not all women will experience hot flashes. These episodes could be experienced prior to, or during the early stages of menopausal transition.

Hot flashes are characterized by the feeling of warmth which originates from the head and the neck area. These episodes, which can happen any time before or during the onset of menopause, can last anywhere from 30 seconds to a few minutes at a time. The experience of hot flashes is different for each woman. It was once believed that women would only experience hot flashes for a few years. But more recent data refutes this belief and shows that women may actually have hot flashes for longer periods than once supposed.

Studies carried out at the University of Pennsylvania have shown that the average duration of hot flashes in a woman is about 4.9 years. However, the study also revealed that up to a third of women would continue to experience hot flashes for up to 10 years. In another study conducted by Women Across the Nation (SWAN), found that women experiences an average of 7.4 years of hot flashes with an average of 4.5 years after the last menstrual period experienced.

Causes of Hot Flashes

The aging process of a woman is a complex shift in hormonal balance, and this is when a constant shift in the hormones is detected. A decline in the production of estrogen is noted in a woman who approaches menopause and this is what is thought to be the underlying cause to hot flashes.

The thermoregulation of a woman is believed to be disrupted and is responsible for the heat sensation a woman experiences during a hot flash episode. Thermoregulation is how the body controls body temperature. Although not fully understood, it is understood that the decline of estrogen levels causes the heat sensation a woman experiences.

Hot flashes is a characteristic commonly associated with menopause, however, hot flashes can also be experienced by men. It can also be experienced for conditions other than that of menopause as well. Women who experience hot flashes should get checked for other underlying medical conditions which may be causing the episodes as there are other medical reasons why a woman or perimenopausal age would be experiencing this. Apart from these situations, hot flashes can also be experienced by some individuals who are taking specific sorts of medications.

Chapter Six: Menopause and Its Health Risks

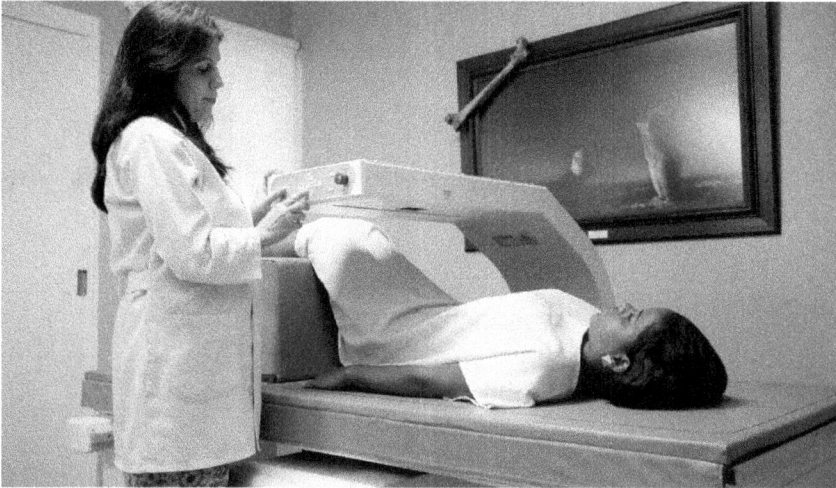

Menopause need not be a time that a woman dreads to see. This is a natural stage in a woman's life much like any other transitional stage she goes through as she matures. If a young girl is prepared for the eventuality of menses and is educated on what she can expect as well as know what her body is capable of doing at this stage in her life, so is menopause a stage she should be inquisitive to learn more of. This is just but a natural stage of the body of a woman. A woman should know what to expect and watch out for in order to lead a better and healthier life.

There are a number of dangers to a woman's health, related to menopause, that a woman should know about in order to empower herself to make better choice and lifestyle changes, if needed. There is a greater risk of heart disease and osteoporosis in menopausal women. Heart disease still remains the leading cause morbidity in America. This is why it is crucial to make certain and determine that your blood work is up to date and healthy.

The levels of cholesterol during the period of menopause may become erratic and fluctuate. This fluctuation causes good cholesterol (or HDL) to decrease as the bad cholesterol (LDL) spikes. These sudden changes and fluctuations could result in a heart attack or a stroke. The decline of the hormone estrogen may also be part to blame, However HRT is not recommended to postmenopausal women to lessen the dangers of this because of the association of HRT with its own health risks, especially to a postmenopausal woman.

Menopause can speed up the development of a bone degenerating disease commonly seen in women.

Osteoporosis is a condition that weakens the bones making the skeletal structure become easily susceptible to damage and breaking. An important component in producing new bone is estrogen. And you have read that estrogen levels in a perimenopausal and menopausal woman is largely decreased. The decrease in the production levels of estrogen during this stage of a woman's life makes her a likely candidate for this bone degenerating disease.

This is why it is important for women to lead healthy lifestyles and exercise on a regular basis whilst they are young. It is imperative and crucial to strengthen your skeletal system early before she reaches the third decade of her life. Preserving a woman's bone density can be achieved by eating foods that contain high amounts of calcium, like milk and dairy products. Another important component to maintaining bone density is Vitamin D because vitamin D is essential for calcium to work.

Osteoporosis

Osteoporosis is a bone disease that results in the deterioration of the bones. It affects the quantity and quality of the bone and results in fracture risks. The bone mineral density typically starts to slow down as a woman ages.

What is concerning is that this decrease in bone density gradually increases during the perimenopausal and menopausal transition. As a result when women hit a certain age and undergo hormonal changes, the result of the menopause transition causes osteoporosis.

The process that leads up to osteoporosis can be silently operating in the background decades before the onset of perimenopause and menopause. Women are usually not aware of this condition until such a time they suffer from a painful fracture.

Treatment Aims of Osteoporosis

The aim of treating osteoporosis is to prevent bone fractures by retarding bone loss whilst increasing bone density and strength. Early detection of osteoporosis can definitely lessen the dangers of later fracture. It is important to note that the treatments available today are not the main cure for this condition. This is why prevention of osteoporosis, through exercise, healthy diet and proper bone maintenance is as important as treatment.

Treatment and Prevention of Osteoporosis

To avoid the debilitating pain of bone degeneration due to osteoporosis, a woman will need to make some lifestyle changes. These changes would include quitting cigarette smoking, limiting or totally avoiding alcohol intake, picking up a smart exercise habit, and eating a balanced diet complete with the appropriate amount of calcium and vitamin D.

Women who do not have sufficient quantities of Calcium and vitamin D supplements may be given recommendation by their gyne to add these as supplement to their diet. There are also available medications that halt bone loss and increase bone strength as it increases bone formation.

Cardiovascular Disease

Heart disease is the leading cause of death in both men and women in the U.S. Before the onset of menopause, women are at a decreased risk of heart disease and stroke as compared with men. This drastically changes around the time of menopause when a woman's risk of cardiovascular disease increases.

The number of coronary heart diseases in postmenopausal women take a significant spike at a rate of two to three times higher compared to women of similar age who have not yet reached the menopause stage.

The increased risk of cardiovascular disease with women in menopause may be associated to the body's decline in the production of the hormone estrogen. In light of other factors, it is ill advised for a postmenopausal woman to take hormone therapy as a preventive measure in order to decrease their risk of heart attack or stroke.

Pelvic Organ Prolapse

When a woman is younger, her pelvic muscles do the necessary, and that is to keep your reproductive organs in their proper place. However, after menopause those muscles that help contain everything where they should be, weakens. Weak pelvic muscles cause the bladder, the vagina, the uterus, or the rectum, to weaken and sag. There are severe cases when compromised parts of a woman's reproductive system can poke out and hang out of the body. The protruding part can rub against clothing which in turn can cause bleeding, severe pain at the most, and discomfort at the very least. When this is the case it can be painfully challenging to empty the bladder or bowels.

Observation and patient reports have shown that women who deliver via natural birth have a higher likelihood to develop pelvic organ prolapse. Those who are highly susceptible to these are those who gave birth naturally, or those who gain excessive during the time of transition. The extra weight can bear down on the floor or the pelvis, putting unwanted pressure on her pelvic organs.

A lot of women put off treatment because of confusion and embarrassment therefore suffer unnecessarily through what is not only painful but also uncomfortable. Women are encouraged to take control of their bodies and take up exercise early. There are about 41 to 51 % of women who suffer from some degree of pelvic organ prolapse.

Pelvic organ prolapse can be determined in a couple of ways. Make an appointment to see your doctor immediately if there is a bulge between the patient's legs or if the complain of having trouble completely emptying the bowels or bladder.

You will want to seek out a specialist who is experienced in this field of women's health to be given the best possible care and treatment. Milder forms of pelvic organ prolapse may not have to have surgical intervention, instead the patient may be recommended to do pelvic floor exercises like Kegels. This is a pelvic floor strengthening exercise where the levator muscles are contracted and held for a five-second count then released for another five seconds. This is done in a number of repetitions. Kegels also assists in controlling and correcting urinary incontinence as preparation for or recovery treatments from natural childbirth.

In more advanced or severe cases the patient may have to undergo surgery or a get pessary. This is a device that a patient with pelvic organ prolapse wears internally. This small medical device that looks like the outer ring of a diaphragm is inserted into the vagina either to treat an infection or to act as support to the uterus and/or other pelvic organs that may need support.

Chapter Seven: Other Health Risks

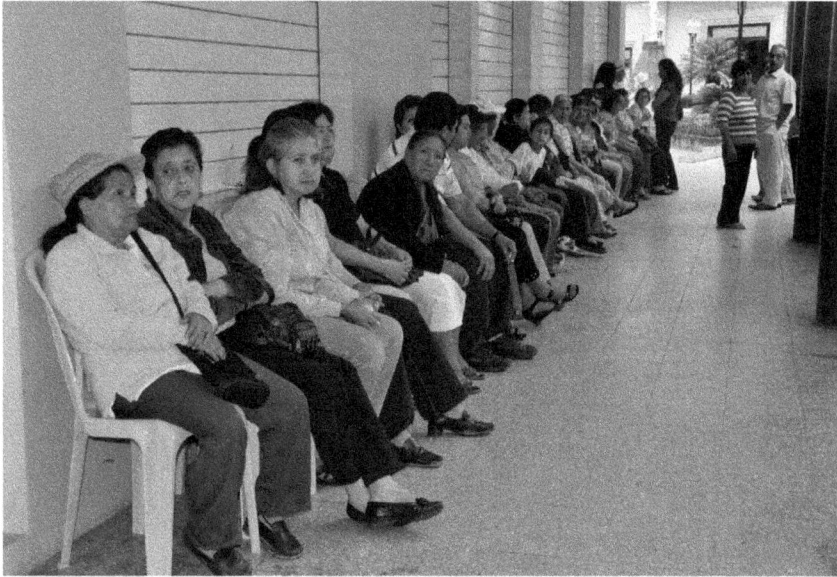

The body make up of a woman is a fascinating but complicated one. It is a vessel that not only carries and incubates a fetus, but it gives birth to a child. It is crucial to know the possible effects of the symptoms of perimenopause and menopause to be able to take decisive action on living healthier lives as well as forming an active lifestyle. The chances of a woman living a good quality of life increases exponentially only if she takes the initiative on setting herself up for a more comfortable, more tolerable experience of perimenopause and menopause. More importantly, better awareness of the implications and effects of her changing body helps empower her to make better health choices.

Liver Disease

During the years of youth when we are young and healthy, our liver has a tendency to easily repair itself from damage caused by substances like alcohol, from infections, or even unnecessary weight. Instead of the body manufacturing healthy cells, during this time of reparation, the liver creates connective tissue.

It appears that estrogen interferes with this process that when the hormone levels fall during menopause, the scar tissue can start to accumulate and over time, this may lead to advanced chronic liver disease. Since estrogen may also have a part in protecting the mitochondria, or your cell's' powerhouses that lie in your liver cells, the decline of the estrogen can ensue damage and further accelerate the aging of the liver.

Take a proactive step and discuss this with your doctor. Take it further and ask your doctor to order a liver enzyme test the next time they order a routine blood test.

Knowing early on if there are elevated levels of the enzyme in your system will allow you and your doctor to take proactive, protective steps. High levels are usually the first indication that there is something amiss with this critical organ. Liver disease is a fairly silent illness that can go unnoticed for years until it becomes more apparent in the advanced stages. Make it a point to take charge of what you can and help yourself along by taking precautionary measures. Women who were born between 1945 and 1965, should also request to be tested for hepatitis C. Hepatitis C is a virus that can wreak horrible havoc on the liver.

Autoimmune Disorders

Feeling tired, moody, and experiencing hot flashes are all normal menopausal symptoms. However, these symptoms could also be indications of an autoimmune disorder. Autoimmune disorders can come in the form of multiple sclerosis, lupus, or rheumatoid arthritis according to medical experts on reproductive endocrinology and infertility at Johns Hopkins University School of Medicine.

Get yourself checked out because the fatigue, hot flashes and moodiness could be a new immune problem cropping up at the time of menopause. On the other hand, the change of life (coming into menopause) might cause a condition you already had to worsen. The changes in this estrogen hormone may result to excessive inflammation in the patient's body and may cause certain body systems to turn on themselves.

Make sure that you keep close tabs and track any symptoms you undergo during menopause. Make it a point to list these down and discuss them with your doctor during your next checkup. If a woman knows that they already have an autoimmune issue, she will need to make sure to express this to her doctor. Explain and detail what you're going through to your rheumatologist and/or endocrinologist, in addition to your gynecologist. Your physician's are your partners in finding solutions and remedies. They can help you keep tabs on your disease and tweak your treatment as necessary.

Dry Eye

Menopause may leave you feeling dry in the most unwanted and unexpected places. Another little-known symptom of menopause is the dry eye syndrome that affects about 61 % of women in the perimenopausal and menopausal stages. And just like other symptoms of menopause, it is the hormones that are to blame. Dropping hormone levels affect the composition of tears in the eyes as well as the ocular tissues.

Symptoms of dry eyes include:

- Light sensitivity
- Dryness
- Blurred vision
- Burning sensations
- Gritty and sandy sensation

Most people are aware that men and women create hormones. It is known that women predominantly create estrogen as men create testosterone. But, what some people don't know is that both men and women can create both hormones-just on different manufacturing levels.

Testosterone, typically thought of as the male hormone, plays a vital role in the function of the meibomian glands. The meibomian glands produces oily film which helps in preserving the fluids that keep the eyes lubricated.

When the production of testosterone declines, this oily layer will tend to get thinner, allowing for more water to evaporate from the eyes. This then leaves behind irritating salt, ultimately resulting in discomfort in the eyes. In addition, the cells of the lacrimal glands, the glands which produce antibodies which protect the surface of the eyes, start to fail a lot faster after menopause.

This may explain why women of an advanced age suffer more serious conditions related to sight and the eyes as compared to their counterparts. These symptoms of dry, scratchy, burning eyes can be troublesome but, can often are treated effectively with simple measures leading to major improvements in the quality of life without surgical intervention. Successful treatment hinges on three major strategies like increasing eye lubrication decreasing tear outflow, and reducing eyelid inflammation.

Even those who enjoy 20/20 eyesight should check in with an eye doctor on a scheduled basis, once they reach the age of 40. See an eye specialist as soon as you can and discuss your symptoms to get the correct treatment. The good news is that there are treatments and medications available. A prescription for tear duct plugs to help prevent moisture loss from the eyes should help this situation.

Protect your eyes and avoid environmental triggers by doing what you can with how it affects your eyes. The wind, dry air, as well as pollutants can all play a part and contribute to dried-out eyes. While you can't completely control the world around you, you can take a stance on how much havoc these elements wreck on your eyes.

Again, being proactive in the care of your body as well as its parts which largely falls on you and you should take measures when you can. Take care of your eyes on windy days by wearing glasses or sunglasses. These can help block the wind in your eyes that can prevent it from drying up.

Use a humidifier in your house, this can bring much needed relief for your eyes, and even does wonders for the skin to boot. If you have an air conditioner in your home, changing out or cleaning out the air conditioner's filter can also keep eye-irritating pollutants at bay and prevent from infiltrating the home.

Hearing Loss

Degradation of some of the things we take for granted, like our sense of hearing, often come with age, but more so, apparently for a woman, after menopause. Once again, it is the decrease of hormone production that is to blame. Estrogen plays a vital role in your cochlea; this is the snail-shaped organ located in the inner ear. They help your brain process sounds.

This may sound redundant, and something that your mother might chide, but staying and keeping healthy throughout your life will do advantageous wonders to the body later on, and that includes the ears. A study conducted recently revealed that women who kept an active lifestyle and exercised the most had a 17% reduced risk of suffering from hearing loss.

Another research, published in the American Journal of Clinical Nutrition, showed that women who maintained a good and healthy diet and consumed the adequate amounts of foods rich in beta-carotene displayed less cases of hearing loss as opposed to those who didn't. So, take it upon yourself to eat healthily and keep moving. Make it a point to have a good exercise routine, complemented by smart food choices.

Sleep Apnea

Sleeping problem arise from the time of perimenopause to after the onset of menopause (postmenopause) and these include the much talked about hot flashes when one is awakened in the middle of the night drenching in sweat, only to find it difficult to go back to sleep. Mood disorders that come along with the shifts in hormone levels are also culprit to keeping women up at night plagued with worry and anxiety.

It is in the knowing that one can take charge of what they face and how they tackle it. Not only are these some of the disturbances caused by the changes of perimenopause and post - menopause, generally, females are 3.5 times likelier to suffer sleep apnea as compared to before the transition.

This is a sleep disorder that causes a person to temporarily cease taking natural breaths whilst asleep. Not only does this sleep disorder cause sleep interruption resulting in the feeling of not having a good restful sleep,

sleep apnea also raises the possibilities of developing more serious health conditions.

A woman has a higher tendency to suffer from sleep apnea after menopause because the progesterone in the respiratory system diminishes.

With age, the skin in the neck also wears thin, which may impinge on the airway, causing the obstruction of nighttime breathing. The weight gain during menopause and the extra fat accumulated in the wrong places can obstruct the ability to breathe easily and the respiratory system as well.

Seek out a sleep specialist if you're suffering from sleep apnea. You will want to reach out and consult the expertise of an expert in sleep disorder. Loud snoring is one sign of sleep apnea; many women later discover that it is sleep apnea that is the culprit of their sleeplessness. Having the sensation of wanting to go to sleep during the day, is one more reason why you should go to the doctor's office.

One treatment you may want to discuss with your physician is a CPAP. This is a dental device that helps a person breath comfortably whilst asleep.

Chapter Eight: Diet and Nutrition for Women

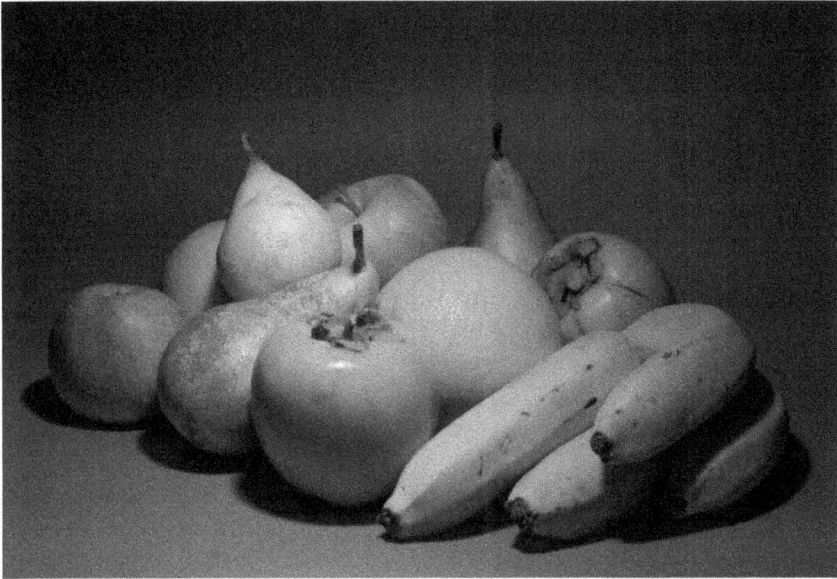

The whole theme of this book revolves around one thing, and it is the importance of keeping healthy and eating right for a better, future you. Adding the correct and appropriate foods to your diet as one approaches menopause can in fact, lessen, limit or prevent symptoms of menopause later in life. The earlier a woman makes healthy dietary choices and changes, the easier it may be for them to weather the transition to menopause.

As mothers to daughters, make it your mission to discuss these eventful changes to your young daughters. Just as you did with explaining menstrual period, sex and the effects of sex (pregnancy,, STD's), so should menopause be a part of your scheduled life-talks with your daughters.

In any case, it is a woman's responsibility to find out about her body. Menopause may seem like a period in a woman's life when she would feel as if her body were giving out on her, literally and in reality. Many of the symptomatic signs of other conditions can be attributed to the changes in a maturing woman's body. It is up to you as a woman to find out what you are up against to form the correct dietary and habits early on or at the very least, take back the reign and make the necessary adjustments to your lifestyle now.

It is true that some of the symptoms of menopause can be downright bothersome, to say the least. Dry skin can be remedied with adequate moisturizing and hot flashes can be aided along with cooling devices and lighter clothing. However there are more concerning diseases and conditions, such as bone loss and cardiovascular diseases, that a woman becomes susceptible to when she reaches the age of menopause. These are even made more pronounced by the longer period of perimenopause when a woman would start to experience many of the symptoms more vividly.

It is therefore important to form a habit of healthy eating early in life. If you are a young mother, setting this good example early in your growing daughter's life will help her make the correct food choices as she prepares for adulthood.

If you haven't exactly been eating healthy or consciously choosing healthy and beneficial foods for your wellbeing, now is a time to start. If you are a mother of a young girl nearing her teens, make it a point to start serving up healthier food fares that will become the foundation of your young daughter's health. A good, balanced diet is beneficial to all human beings and needs to be a priority in order to get the best out of health and out of life.

Knowing the right kind of foods to eat to help along the symptoms of menopause is essential. The earlier (or sooner) these foods become regular food increases one's chances of being fit for the later years in life.

Water

Make it a point to drink eight glasses of water a day, in proper intervals. Drinking the correct amount of water can help maintain the skin's moisture and offset dryness.

With the proper amount of water in your system, you will be able to help along and stave off the dryness of the vagina; a common complaint of women going through menopause. Water also helps moisturize the skin, another noticeable change as a woman goes through menopause.

Consuming the appropriate amount of water helps relieve and avoid bloating in women who experience hormonal changes. This symptom is commonly seen some time before menstrual life of the individual ends for good.

This period is called perimenopause, and is equally important to know about.

Calcium

The calcium needs of a maturing woman increases during the period of menopause due to the loss of estrogen. The decrease of this important hormone contributes to bone degradation. A woman not on an estrogen replacement therapy must consume the necessary amount of calcium to prevent the deterioration of the bones.

If a woman does take hormone replacement therapy she must aim for 1,000 milligrams of calcium each day. This can be difficult for many women to achieve through diet alone. So you will need to consider a combination of calcium-rich foods in your diet, and supplement it with milk and nonfat yogurt, along with OTC or prescribed calcium supplements.

Vitamin D

A woman who is in the perimenopause and menopause stages will have to get enough vitamin D. This is critical to the bone protection of the woman. One natural source of vitamin D is the sun. However, experts agree that it is crucial for the health of the woman. Vitamin D is therefore highly recommended for woman who is in the perimenopausal and menopausal stage. This is especially true during winter time.

Doctors recommend that women in menopause get anywhere from 1,000 to 2,000. Every woman is different so it is best to discuss your actual dose intake with your specialist.

Fruits and Vegetables

The metabolism slows down as people get older, and many women in their mid-forties have a tendency to lead more sedentary, less active lifestyles. This all equates and results to weight gain, and one of the most dreaded of all menopause symptoms (at least by the standards of women).

Load up on crisp veggies and fresh fruits that are low in calorie needed to stay healthy while keeping off the weight. Many fruits and vegetables also give great benefits to the biggest organ of the body, the skin! Fruits and vegetables have been long known for their beneficial advantages in the proper portions and balance. They also do wonders for the digestive system

Whole Grains

There are some whole grains, like quinoa, barley, steel-cut oatmeal, and brown rice, which provide essential B vitamins. These foods help boost an individual's energy, they help manage stress, and in addition, whole grain foods keep the digestive system functioning optimally. Found in whole grains are essentials like folic acid. This greatly helps in lowering the risk of cardiovascular diseases, many of which arises once the woman reaches menopause.

Iron

A woman will need to limit her iron intake when nearing her perimenopausal years and most especially, upon reaching menopause. Iron needs to decrease during the menopausal years, therefore, be mindful that you eat a good balance of dairy products, grains and lean protein; these should supply the right amount of iron in your diet if calculated correctly. Unless your doctor prescribes iron supplement, avoid taking OTC multivitamins or iron pills.

Soy

Some experts would recommend soy for to help relieve symptoms of hot flashes. The results are inconclusive, but word is in that a majority of women swear to the benefits soy has given them toward managing hot flashes since these soy compounds work much like estrogen in the body would.

A study concentrated in Asia showed the advantages of soy in a menopausal woman's diet. They primarily get their soy intake from food which is a staple that comes in various forms. From soft, hard, curds, puddings, to milk, soy can come in a variety of forms and is easy to prepare and mix in dishes.

Some women could either be concerned about the effects of HRT on them, most especially is they had not started the therapy younger. The results define a higher risk of HRT when taken by postmenopausal women to help relieve them of hot flashes.

Young soybean, tofu, tempeh, and edamame are good sources of soy. Look up recipes online since tofu is a good source of other vitamins needed by the body. Keep it natural and stay away from *anything that is processed soy.* Any time a woman can add and make plant-based foods staples to their diet brings great health benefits.

Flaxseed

Rich in omega-3 goodness is flaxseed. Make sure to choose ground flaxseed and not the flaxseed oil. Research has revealed that 40 grams of ground flaxseed each day, can give the similar effects of hormone therapy that can help alleviate and improve the symptoms of menopause like night sweats and hot flashes. Mix in this omega-3 rich food to your everyday food to help ease constipation. It helps keep your blood vessels in good shape.

Low - Calorie Foods

In reality and in terms of the upkeep of good health, calorie intake needs to reduce as we get older. The goal is to eat healthy food that will not contribute to the individual gaining weight. Weight retention in more mature women has been noted, not only because of the sedentary lifestyles most women lead. Even the busiest woman may often times, find themselves bound to a desk only to be freed temporarily to walk to the car where she spends a good part of her day driving from one seat to another.

How well a woman manages the symptoms of menopause later in life will also depend on weight. A woman, who is able to maintain a certain, healthy weight, will be able to better manage the symptoms of menopause.

It is worth adopting and forming a habit of a low fat diet consisting of healthy foods which should include a generous daily amount of healthy foods, in adequate ratios and servings. Do not neglect to have a good exercise habit that will help keep off the poundage.

What to Avoid

Women in the perimenopausal and menopause stage are strongly recommended to avoid consuming sweetened foods, drinking alcohol or taking in caffeine in any form because all of these foods can trigger and set off hot flashes. These can also contribute to the increase bone loss.

Those who are able to manage these symptoms with grace have come to accept this change in their lives as part of their womanhood.

Rather than dreading the day, shrugging it off and ignoring the inevitable, women with foresight and those who intend on enjoying the best out of life will find ways that will help her attain those goals.

Knowing what to expect from menopause allows women to prepare their bodies and minds by not only getting to know what to expect, they too, shall do what is necessary to prepare their bodies and minds by toughening up for the expected.

Many women are expected to rear, raise and care for people in the family, whether they be their children or their elderly parents. From mothers taking care of the family, the kids and their needs, to taking care of aging parents, women have a lot on their plate that it can be easy to overlook the one person doing all these things for the family around them. This is the perfect time and opportunity to look in the mirror and take notice of the one that needs to be cared for as well - yourself. You need to take care of yourself now so you can have the kind of life you want.

Here is a short list of foods and vitamins to take each day for a better nutrition:

- 9 milligrams of iron each day

- You will have to include approximately 21 milligrams of fiber to your diet each day

- 1 ½ cups of fruit

- 2 cups of vegetables

- Drink plenty of water - at least 8 to 10 glasses interspersed throughout the day

- Cut back on fatty food intake

- Limit all sugar and salt intake

- Read and understand food labels

- Menopause and Weight Gain

The lack of estrogen in a menopausal woman is reason for weight gain. It may also contribute to the body becoming less effective. When this happens, this increases fat storage and makes it challenging for the woman to lose weight. Make it a habit to have a routine exercise regimen. Regular physical activity is crucial for the health at any given age, and is especially so for a woman as she transitions to menopause.

During this transitional period of a woman, her metabolism slows down. When this happens, it makes it harder for a woman shed the pounds or keeps on the weight.

Two important components of an effective exercise program for a woman in the perimenopausal stage and at the onset of menopause; aerobic exercise helps the cardio system while resistance workouts help maintain bone strength. A regular exercise regimen can also help to keep unwanted weight off and help elevate the woman's mood. There is no time like now to make lifestyle choices and changes that will promote a better life and a better you.

Chapter Nine: Treatment and Medication

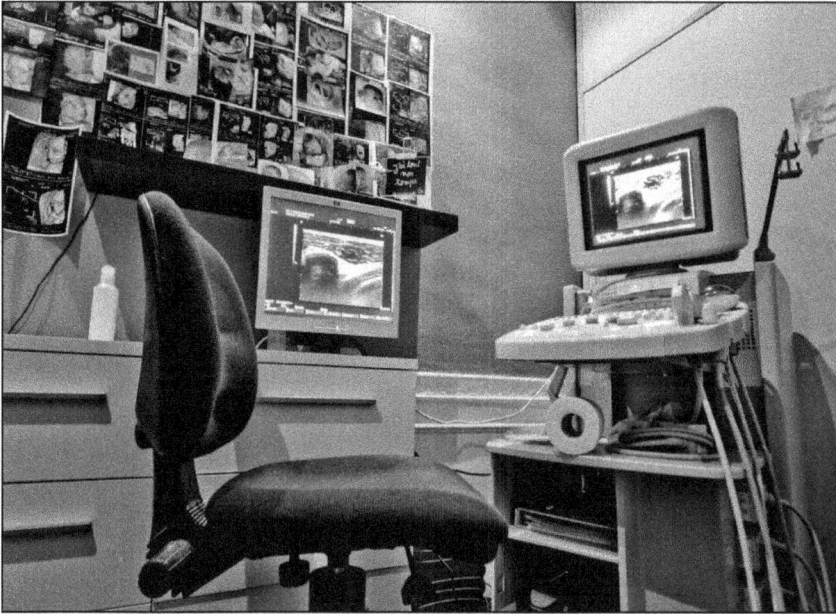

Menopause is not a disease to be dreaded. It is also not a process but a period in a woman's life when she has lost the ability to ovulate. The period before menopause is when she would feel the many of the symptoms that come along with the shift. As much as it is something that will naturally come in a woman's life, it can also come with a host of medical challenges that you can better manage if you were aware. One can tell if they are menopausal if they have gone a whole year without menstruating. The symptoms of menopause occur years before the final period of the woman. For some women perimenopausal symptoms cease to occur a few months after the last period. Others could continue to experience symptoms for a few years after the fact.

The experience of symptoms of perimenopause as well as menopause, are different for each woman. It is important to remember that every woman will experience varying symptoms as well as its intensity. Each woman's experience is highly individual so getting advice from another woman who experiences could be totally different from yours would be futile. Treatments given are customized for each individual.

Menopause is a natural process of a woman's body. However, menopause can trigger drastic changes, not only to the woman's body but also to her mental and emotional state. And because of the drop of estrogen levels, symptoms like depression, mood swings and cognitive changes are some of the issues a woman has to deal with. This is why it is important for women to know what they can do so that they are not caught unawares with the changes in their bodies and chemical makeup.

There are no treatments needed for menopause. However in some cases, menopause may aggravate certain conditions therefore some women are given medication to help along these conditions.

Menopause Treatment: Hormone Therapy

Hormone therapy is administered to women to help in regulating menopause. This kind of treatment is made up of estrogen, or a combination of both estrogen and progesterone. It is administered to the patient by way of pill, patch, or spray. The extended use of HT is ill-advised. In some women, hormone therapy can be detrimental to their overall wellness, making a select few more susceptible to deadly diseases. Therefore, hormone therapy should not to be taken without the knowledge and approval of your physician.

It is therefore recommended that women who are given this therapy to replace estrogen, be given the smallest amount of hormones that are effective to controlling the symptoms that come along with menopause. Make it a point that this therapy be taken for the shortest length of time possible. There are various types of hormone therapies that are available. Your doctor is the best person who can suggest the best solution, and he/she can further determine if you require this treatment.

There is data which suggests that hormone replacement therapy (HRT) could help alleviate symptoms of dry eyes, but a study made up of 25,665 women, revealed a spike in the tendency to dry eye syndrome in women who are on HRT therapy, and especially estrogen. The jury is still out on the exact role and association of HRT to the dry eye syndrome.

HRT once was seen as heaven sent and was thought to help greatly in dousing bouts of hot flashes. However, a major new study lead by the Women's Health Initiative (WHI) has revealed a very disturbing data. WHI researchers, in July 2002, reported that the long-term use of one of the most commonly used HRT preparation, a combination of estrogen and progestin, could promote the increase of a woman's risk of invasive breast cancer, heart disease and stroke. However the risk is seen to be higher in women who started HRT at the onset of menopause as opposed to those women who started HRT way before menopause.

HT is still the most effective way to treat and control the symptoms of menopause. A study of an estrogen-only group, showed no increase or decrease in the occurrence of heart disease. However, those on estrogen-only hormone therapy did manifest a slightly increased risk of stroke.

On its own, estrogen therapy has also been associated with an increased risk of developing endometrial cancer, this is the sort of cancer that attacks the lining of the uterus. Studies show that women who took estrogen therapy may have higher risks of experiencing stroke rather than breast cancer/ hear – attack. As a result, the search for a non-drug approach to managing menopausal symptoms has accelerated.

Bioidentical Hormone Therapy

Bioidentical hormone therapy is the term that has been used to refer to hormones gleaned from plants. These are prepared to tailor fit the individual requirements of each patient at compounding pharmacies. An increasing interest, in recent years, has been noticed in the mention and use of was termed as bioidentical hormone therapy, which is aimed to treat the perimenopausal symptoms of women. Bioidentical hormone concocted preparations and medications that contain hormones.

These hormones possess the same chemical formula like the ones produced by the body naturally with the difference being that these hormones are made through human and scientific intervention using natural resources that are tweaked. Some of these bioidentical hormone preparations have the FDA stamp of approval and are produced by drug companies. Then there are those which are made at compounding pharmacies. These are special drugstores that measure and lay out preparations, specifically suited for each patient. They are manufactured with the patient's needs in consideration. Compounded products are not standardized and are not FDA approved preparations. They come in cream or gels forms and are typically administered through transdermal.

Advocates of BHRT believe that their use of these compounded concoctions may help them dodge ill effects that are associated with the use of synthetic hormones. Studies to support this do not claim medical effectivity nor have they been tested by governing medical institutions.

The decision on whether to take hormone therapy, or bioidentical HRT is an individual decision. Both patient and doctor will need to strongly consider the pros and cons.

Current recommendation on the use of hormone therapy dictates these to be used at the smallest, most effective doses. It is also recommended to not use this for too long and that HRT only be utilized if the advantages outweigh the disadvantages for the woman.

Antidepressant medications have been prescribed to some women to help control some symptoms of menopause.

Medications associated with SSRIs have shown to be effective in managing the symptoms of hot flashes in up to 60% of women. However, some antidepressant medications may be associated with side effects, including decreased libido or sexual dysfunction. Other prescription medications have shown to offer some relief for hot flashes, although their specific purpose is not the treatment of hot flashes.

All of these therapies and treatments may have side effects, so make sure you discuss the use of these with your physician prior to using them. Your doctor will need to sign off and approve any drug or treatment.

Often prescribed to women in perimenopause are oral contraceptives which have HRT components. Oral contraceptives can help treat irregular vaginal bleeding. Before commencing with treatment, the physician must first figure out the cause of the bleeding. Menopausal women experience considerable blood loss when they are on estrogen.

The list of contraindications of pills experiencing the transition of menopause is similar to those for pre - menopausal women. Locally applied hormone and non-hormone treatments are hormonal treatments meant to address the lack of estrogen. Creams and moisturizing lotions applied to the vaginal area as well as using lubricants during intercourse, are non-hormonal options that assist in alleviating the irritating and uncomfortable sensation of dry skin. Betadine, when topically applied on the outer parts of the vaginal area, could help in relieving the symptoms of vaginal discomfort.

Chapter Ten: Herbal Supplements to Ease Menopause Symptoms

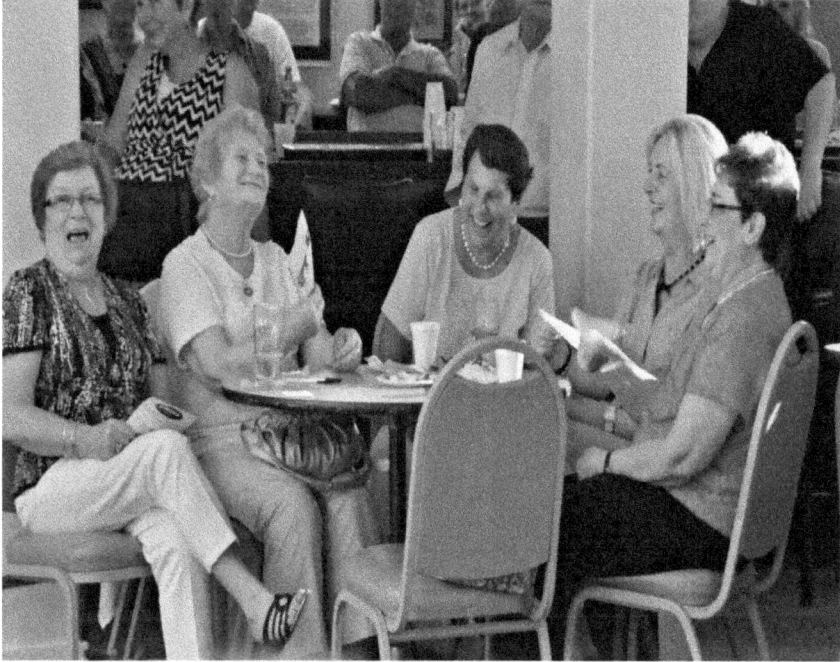

Many women and doctors turn to natural remedies in order to avoid the side effects of pharma manufactured drugs. There are certain herbal medicines and botanicals that are lauded in the treatment and management of hot flashes and symptoms. However, the Food and Drug Administration doesn't regulate herbal supplements, so effectiveness or safety cannot always be guaranteed.

Good Nutrition and Food Supplements

Women are encouraged to take charge of their bodies and take the necessary measures to prepare for this natural occurrence in the lives of women. Start leading a healthy lifestyle. Make sure that you get your routine checkups done. These checkups should check on your blood pressure cholesterol, and blood sugar.

- Do go in for scheduled mammograms

- Consume plant - based foods that have plant estrogens as these may help in slightly increasing estrogen levels

- Soy helps relieve symptoms of menopause.

- Make sure that you get enough calcium and iron. Both of these components are crucial to the wellness of menopausal women

- Work with your doctor so that you can create a
  suitable health plan which would include a nutritious
  diet, the proper amount and the correct sort of
  physical activity, as well as improving cognitive
  skills.

Plant estrogens have shown great promise and
effectiveness in managing the symptoms of menopause.
These plants have Isoflavones chemical compounds that are
usually found soy as well as plant-derived estrogens. These
plants - based products have a chemical structure that is
similar to the estrogens that's naturally produced in the
body though of course, their effectiveness is not as high
compared to the natural estrogens.

There are two types of isoflavones, called genistein
and daidzein, which are found in soybeans, lentils and
chickpeas. These are considered to be the strongest estrogens
of the phytoestrogens.

Research has revealed these compounds to help
alleviate and relieve hot flashes and other symptoms of
menopause. Women who have had breast cancer and do not
wish to take hormone therapy with estrogen resort to the use
of soy products to find relief from menopausal symptoms.
Many women perceive that plant estrogens are natural
remedies and are therefore safer than hormone therapy, but
this has yet to be proven scientifically. .

Vitamin E

Some women have reported that their intake of
vitamin E supplements has helped alleviate some symptoms
of menopause. There are those who report that vitamin E
can give relief from mild hot flashes. However scientific
studies are still lacking which is why there's still not enough
evidence to support that vitamin E may relieve symptoms of
menopause.

Black Cohosh

This is a herbal preparation which has been widespread in Europe. It is said to bring relief against hot flashes. This herb has currently been gaining popularity in the U.S. Further studies and research is still underway to determine the effectiveness and safety of black cohosh.

Other alternative therapies for menopause symptoms include supplements and substances which have been marketed as natural treatments against the symptoms of menopause. Some of these products include dong quai, licorice, chaste berry, and wild yam. However, as with other herbal supplements, scientific studies have yet to prove the safety of the Black Cohosh.

Should you want to try these remedies, or other herbal products, you will want to initially discuss this with your doctor since there are some botanical supplements that can interact adversely with prescription drugs.

Treatment for Severe Menopause Symptoms

Hormone therapy has been said to be effective in helping alleviate many of the troublesome symptoms of menopause. Taking low doses of contraceptive pills is one option for perimenopausal women to help with irregular vaginal bleeding as well as relieve the symptoms of hot flashes, whilst local vaginal hormone treatments can be applied directly to the vagina as a treatment of symptoms brought about by vaginal estrogen deficiency.

Celebrating Menopause

A lot of women has embraced this natural shift in their lives and live better because of it. Menopause need not be a time to dread. It is not a topic that needs to be shoved way back only to be dealt with when it is apparent. Menopause need not be a dirty word or the butt of jokes. Celebrate the new phase of your womanhood.

The transition through menopause can have many advantages if you know how to look at the bigger picture.

You will not have to suffer through the inconvenience of monthly periods or deal with the painful and sometimes disorienting symptoms of PMS. You will also be able to enjoy sex without having to think about getting knocked up.

Spend time on you and love yourself. Use this time to rediscover yourself, life and what else it has to offer. It is also a great time to bring the spark back into the bedroom and to rediscover your body and the, still, many advantages that are ahead of you.

Photo Credits

Page 11 Photo by userGreenFlames09 via Flickr.com,

https://www.flickr.com/photos/greenflames09/132172081/in/photostream/

Page 21 Photo by user Stephen Melkisethian via Flickr.com,

https://www.flickr.com/photos/stephenmelkisethian/12391486435/

Page 28 Photo by user Ed Uthman via Flickr.com,

https://www.flickr.com/photos/euthman/2722043681/

Page 34 Photo by userKaren P via Flickr.com,

https://www.flickr.com/photos/karenpaulson/1607212314/

Page 44 Photo by user Neil Moralee via Flickr.com,

https://www.flickr.com/photos/neilmoralee/8105981360/

Page 58 Photo by user PresidenciaRD via Flickr.com,

https://www.flickr.com/photos/presidenciard/37766304896/

Page 63 Photo by userMunicipioPinas via Flickr.com,

https://www.flickr.com/photos/municipiopinas/4639350589/

Page 78 Photo by user Keith Williamson via Flickr.com,

https://www.flickr.com/photos/elwillo/8169824956/

Page 91 hoto by user Mitch Huang via Flickr.com,

https://www.flickr.com/photos/mitch98000/4343345869/

Page 100 Photo by user Jeff Meade via Flickr.com,

https://www.flickr.com/photos/irishphiladelphia/1497787001
6/

References

"Treating Menopause's Secret Symptom" – WebMD.com

https://www.webmd.com/women/features/treating-menopauses-secret-symptom#2

"Flaxseed" – WebMD.com

https://www.webmd.com/a-to-z-guides/supplement-guide-flaxseed-oil#1

"Help for Hot Flashes" – WebMD.com

https://www.webmd.com/women/features/soy-hot-flashes

"Menopause and Good Nutrition" – WebMD.com

https://www.webmd.com/menopause/guide/staying-healthy-through-good-nuitrition#1

"The Surprising Ways Menopause Can Lead to Hearing Loss" - BottomlineInc.com

https://bottomlineinc.com/health/menopause/the-surprising-ways-menopause-can-lead-to-hearing-loss

"Menopause and Dry Eyes: The Surprising Connection" - HuffingtonPost.com

https://www.huffingtonpost.com/ellen-sarver-dolgen/dry-eyes_b_3769248.html

"Premature & early menopause" - JeanHailes.org.au

https://jeanhailes.org.au/health-a-z/menopause/premature-early-menopause

"Dealing with Early Menopause" - HealthLine.com

https://www.healthline.com/health/menopause/dealing-early#diagnosis

"Premature Menopause Symptoms, Causes, and Treatments" - Medicinenet.com

https://www.medicinenet.com/premature_menopause_medical_procedural_causes/article.htm#signs_and_symptoms_of_early_menopause

"What are the complications and effects of menopause on chronic medical conditions?" - Medicinenet.com

https://www.medicinenet.com/premature_menopause_medical_procedural_causes/article.htm

"Menopause" - Medicinenet.com

https://www.medicinenet.com/menopause/article.htm#what_are_the_complications_and_effects_of_menopause_on_chronic_medical_conditions